STOP

SNORING

TAKE BACK YOUR NIGHT

ZITA RATH

Table of Contents

This page was left blank intentionally

Who Needs to Read this?

If you are reading this, there is a good probability that one or both of you, as well as the person you spend your evenings with or someone you care about, snores. Losing sleep has serious negative effects. When a wall of noise stands between you and the sleep you so desperately need and deserve each night, it may make you feel a little insane.

You're looking for a solution, which is why you're reading this. You don't want to snore any longer, and your sleeping companion has to quit as well. Please do not assume that this is a brochure for snore-resolving surgery. This book offers several really simple treatments that, in addition to completely eliminating snoring, have also been shown to be lifesaving. These non-surgical options will help you get the rest you need, whether you snore or you sleep next to someone who does. Either way, there will be more good sleep available.

Prior to moving on, it is important to comprehend the physical causes of snoring and its most fundamental causes. We can examine snoring's problematic nature in more detail after we have a better understanding of how it functions. At this point, we'll examine the detrimental impacts of snoring, as well as what it means for the human body.

When we are aware of what snoring is and what it can indicate, we can go on to finding a solution. Understanding surgical methods is important when looking for biological process remedies since it explains how and why choosing this approach to treat snoring is hazardous and often ineffective.

By the time you've finished reading, your opinion of snoring will have significantly altered; no one you care about or yourself will find it amusing or acceptable.

INTRODUCTION

Snoring is not only annoying. Snoring is a symptom, a representation of harm brought on by an underlying problem, not merely something that individuals do. Even today, most individuals still fail to detect the harm caused by snoring since it has long been mistakenly believed to be a normal feature of many, if not most, people's sleeping patterns.

What Damage Is There?

The restorative process that we need to experience in order to be healthy and alert is sleep. Snoring is an annoyance that may keep us from falling asleep, keep us from breathing comfortably, and even keep us awake due to the noise it might make. Snoring is not simply an issue that the snorer has to cope with; it may have an impact on everyone around, particularly a bed partner or someone who shares a room.

A person who must share a bed or sleeping space with someone who snores may find it impossible to obtain a good night's sleep due to the snoring of the other person. Snoring creates more issues than just noise. People die from sleep apnea, not snoring, in its most harmful form. Snoring is the only audible form of sleep apnea, or when a person unintentionally pauses breathing while sleeping. A snorer's excessively loud and heavy breathing is caused by sleep apnea.

A person who has sleep apnea often changes positions in the middle of the night or wakes up gasping. A person's mood, temperament, and capacity for concentration and attention, as well as their ability to be an effective member of society, are all negatively impacted by a chronic lack of deep sleep. How terrible can it be? Snoring is sometimes portrayed as charming or comical in the sense of how absurd a person's snoring may be. However, let's see how amusing you would find it if you were in that situation.

Consider it a gift in your life if you have never had to share a bed with a snorer. Let's compare the snore's often bombastic sound. The following samples, each of which registers at least as many decibels as the typical snorer, should help you understand what so many people must put up with in order to have a decent night's sleep:

- Using a gas-powered lawnmower;
- Using a shop vacuum
- A motorbike in motion
- A plane traveling slowly
- Using a chainsaw

Your kitchen's appliances are all operating simultaneously.

The important thing to keep in mind about these situations is that you are constantly subjected to them while attempting to acquire rest—deep, uninterrupted, high-quality sleep. This isn't exaggerating; just ask anybody who has slept with a snorer what it's like, and you'll get an earful, so be ready to listen.

Snoring does not go away as quickly as the hiccups do; instead, it persists until anything is done to stop it or the snorer passes away while they are still asleep.

CHAPTER ONE

Recognizing Snoring

Snoring is generally regarded as any form of resonance sound produced by breathing during sleep. Where the mouth and nasal passageways converge, or the crux of the snore, is where breathing during sleep creates vibration, or snoring. Breathing passage restrictions are the cause of this vibration. Since restricted breathing passages are what cause snoring, it should be known that the louder and more bothersome the snoring will be, the more severely restricted these passages are.

The body is in a relaxed, prone posture during sleeping, which is why snoring only happens at that time. The tissues that make up the airway function similarly to muscles. These tissues essentially obstruct the breathing route while a person is laying down since they become slightly flaccid when sleeping. This causes the sleeper to have trouble breathing, which leads to more vigorous breathing, which is then equivalent to snoring.

What Elements Affect a Snorer's Snore Volume?

Each individual is distinct in their physical makeup and composition. This has an impact on why some individuals snore really loudly. The tone and pitch are also components of snoring; essentially, we all have the same elements but each of us has a distinctive voice that is easy to recognize.

The many components involved in this

process will determine how loud a person may snore. Snoring is an audible warning that the body is battling for air because there is essentially a flap of tissue blocking the airway we need to breathe, making breathing more laborious and aggressive to provide our lungs, body, and brain with oxygen. Anyone, including infants, may be impacted by this problem.

The tissue obstructing the airway will vibrate in proportion to the force required to receive the essential oxygen our body is depriving itself of since the narrower the breathing passageways are when we sleep, the more forceful the body will become in an attempt to get the air it requires. Snoring becomes so loud because of this. Most snoring is done by males. In general, men snore more than any other gender.

This is related to the physical makeup of the male body, namely the thicker-than-average neck in this instance. Male necks tend to be fleshier, therefore there is often more tissue within. Of course, the chance of loud snoring increases with the amount of tissue in the neck and the area around the breathing passages.

Progesterone, which is naturally produced by females, acts as a snoring defence. True, some women snore as loudly and violently as men, and in some cases even louder, but it is not as common in women as it is in men. Men who snore are treated with progesterone as a kind of therapy.

Causes and Amplifiers of Snoring

Snoring is a symptom of several conditions, as we've previously mentioned. This symptom appears as a sound that results from the inability to breathe freely when you're sleeping. What, then, is the problem? This annoying condition is not only caused by the tissues used for breathing. Although there are almost twice as many male snorers as there are female snorers, these elements are not gender-specific; they are problems that both men and women face. Our lifestyle and health have a role in snoring;

These elements may be combined in many ways and include the following:

- Allergies often impair breathing.
- Antihistamines dry up the typically wet nasal passages.
- A cold or the flu may also lead to difficult breathing.
- Nasal passage surgery-related tissue scarring.

- The sinuses' overall thickness of the tissues
- Abuse of nasal spray causes sinus and airway irritation.
- Snorting illicit drugs Excessively large tonsils or adenoids
- A goitre is an enlarged thyroid gland. A large tongue

Obesity causes the neck and soft tissues to thicken. A large stomach Utilization of Alcohol Smoking the Aging Men are more likely than women to have some of these problems, such as an excessively large stomach. This is thought to be a contributing factor to why men often have greater snoring issues than women.

Additionally, illicit, over-the-counter, and prescription-controlled medications have been linked to snoring-causing side effects, including nasal dryness and relaxed airway and throat tissues. We have examined what snoring is and deconstructed the physiological mechanism. We have also discussed the many factors that influence and contribute to snoring, so it is time to go a little further to understand the genuinely harmful effects that snoring may have on a person's health.

Why is snoring so bad?

The idea of snoring as a whole is somewhat subversive, and this is where the biggest risk with snoring lies—in how harmless most people think it is. Snoring as a term appears unproblematic, but it is. The word's connotation does not accurately describe what happens when someone snores, which is when their body is oxygen-deprived and has to breathe more forcefully to forcibly open the airway.

Snoring is essentially a silent cry for aid that signals that I am not breathing. Because of this widespread misconception about snoring, individuals find it hard to believe that it might bring emotional problems and health dangers. The intensity of snoring and the many problems it causes are discussed in this section of the book.

The majority of individuals are unaware that, although it is ubiquitous, snoring is neither natural nor healthy. The Physical Aspects of Snoring A shift in perspective, or a dynamic change in what snoring signifies, is necessary before individuals can properly comprehend what it genuinely signifies. Snoring poses serious risks, which cannot be emphasized enough.

The list of physical health problems linked to snoring is condensed here;

- Snore apnea
- Heart Illness
- The stroke
- Migraines Night time sweating
- Acid reflux
- Inflamed limbs
- Deteriorated immune system
- Hearing loss

Remember that there are many more health problems associated with snoring; this is only a partial list. These problems, as well as snoring, are not only a problem for grownups. Snoring affects people of all ages and genders, rendering anyone vulnerable to the many harmful impacts it may have. Let's examine one of the most significant problems associated with snoring in greater detail.

In-Depth Discussion of Sleep Apnea Sleep apnea is a silent killer that strikes in the dead of night when a person is most vulnerable—while they are sleeping. This should be plenty to convince anybody who snores or even cares about someone who snores to look for a solution; discover a means to relieve the problem while sleeping so as to prevent breathing from ceasing entirely. The word apnea, which means lack of breathing, originated in ancient Greek.

Asphyxiation only occurs before sleep apnea. Snoring and sleep apnea are directly related; in fact, snoring is merely another name for sleep apnea. Snoring is a lack of breath caused by tissue obstructing the airway. If the body senses the obstruction and breathes rapidly to clear it, the obstructive tissue will vibrate and produce the sound associated with snoring. Snoring occurs when the body strains to breathe vigorously enough to break the obstruction, but sleep apnea occurs when breathing ceases. The connection is clear.

A person's health might suffer from sleep apnea even if it is not deadly. The oxygen that is absorbed into the lungs and subsequently into the bloodstream during breathing is what the body uses to transport itself. Without breathing, which is what sleep apnea means, our bodies are robbed of the oxygen they need to exist and function to their full potential. An imbalance in the bloodstream brought on by a shortage of oxygen results in too much carbon dioxide being produced.

A hazardous condition brought on by an excess of carbon dioxide in the body may cause heart disease, a stroke, or brain damage.

The Emotional Consequences of Snoring

Snoring has consequences for others as well as the snorer. Anyone who lives next to someone who snores loudly knows this. Just as significant as the health dangers associated with snoring are the effects it has on the people around the snorer. Snoring that is as loud as a motorbike or other internal combustion engine might prevent a companion from falling asleep. Every night, a loud snorer might disturb everyone in the home.

This should start to highlight the wide range

of issues that can develop as a result of snoring. Trying to obtain a full night of deep, undisturbed sleep is a fruitless endeavour for anybody who sleeps next to someone who snores, shares a room with them, or even just resides in the same building. Situations like this may be quite frustrating since the snorer may not be aware of it or may think there is nothing that can be done about it. There is a high emotional cost associated with snoring; a few instances of emotional problems brought on by snoring include: Sleep deprivation may lead to sadness or anxiety.

Relationships, especially marriages, end Removal from a home for annoying tenants Fighting between roommates or neighbours because it disturbs their sleep Due to insufficient sleep, poor performance at work results in unemployment.

Issues with short- and long-term memory brought on by little sleep
A lack of empathy from people who are impacted by snoring.

These are just a few of the many emotional issues that come hand-in-hand with snoring. Snoring has significant negative consequences for people who are exposed to it. The mental feelings related to the person who snores and the one who must cope with it lie under the surface of each of these emotional states. Here are a few of the emotional conditions brought on by snoring:

- o feeling worn out
- o frustration
- o resentment
- o anger
- o lack of initiative

- o feelings of distress
- o desperation
- o perplexity
- o lack of self-esteem

It is simple to see how a lack of sleep might alter one's behaviour, particularly if the lack of sleep was caused by someone else's snoring. When they are the one being kept awake, snorers might soon lose one's sympathy. How, therefore, may the snoring problem be fixed? The surgical technique will be covered first, along with reasons why it shouldn't be the first option, even if there are other schools of thought and methods for treating snoring.

This page was left blank intentionally

CHAPTER TWO

Surgery and snoring

The twenty-first century offers amazing improvements in both medicine and surgery. Since the dawn of time, people have struggled with snoring. In this day and age, snorers are fortunate since the effects of snoring are now beginning to be recognized. Use the resources available from the medical community to learn why you are snoring before trying any method to stop it.

Knowing the underlying reason for your snoring can help you find the best ways to minimize or eradicate it as much as you can. Allergy medications and surgery are also alternatives for alleviation, but the latter is almost never the best option for snoring. Snoring is not usually affected by this. The nature of surgery and snoring actually don't mix that well. For a number of reasons, surgery should be the very last option.

Any surgical procedure has risks, and these risks are frequently outweighed by the benefits; however, this is typically the case when there are few, if any, other options for treating a condition that is affecting a person's health and well-being. Surgery is a process of exploration. Surgery by its very nature seems counterintuitive to treating a problem like snoring, particularly when there are alternative approaches that are considerably less intrusive and may be just as effective.

Surgery results in scarring, and because it is an exploratory process, a doctor cannot predict what they will find until they are actually performing the procedure. The patient is opened and cut. After having a surgery like a rhinoplasty, snoring is frequently the result of the surgery itself.

In reality, a sizable portion of those who have undergone snoring surgeries have reported that they did not always produce the desired outcome. Surgery for snoring is uncommon and less dependable than certain other surgical operations that are regularly carried out. The surgical solution is to remove any extra tissue that may be causing the obstruction, since snoring is the consequence of tissue obstructing the airway.

This may be a sensible and acceptable solution for certain individuals, but it is definitely not the case for the vast majority of snorers. Remember that snoring is often, if not always, a symptom of something else going on in the body rather than the actual cause of the issue. There isn't a one-size-fits-all solution to solve everyone's snoring problem since each person's snoring problem will have a different and unique underlying reason. An illustration of the complexities of snoring and how surgery does not always treat the underlying cause may be found on the following page.

A case in point is insurance. Let's examine something basic and unrelated to medicine: car insurance. Let's look at 20 people who have bad driving records, according to their insurance providers. All of these drivers will experience a $500 premium increase when their insurance is renewed as a result of that questionable distinction.

Now, it may appear from a distance that all of these drivers are in the same situation (or same car, as it were). And based on that supposition, one way to solve this issue might be to just give each of these people an additional $500 in cash. As strange as it may sound, each of these 20 drivers can actually solve this issue by finding an additional $500 to pay their insurance premium, which is what this so-called solution will do.

But is this prudent? No!

Some of those drivers—probably more than a few of them—won't truly make amends for the reasons their insurance provider could label them as poor drivers. They simply won't understand why they drive poorly, and as a result, some of them are likely to continue to be **bad drivers** and pay higher insurance premiums the following year—this time after a few more collisions or tickets.

As you can see, giving each person a nice gift of $500 to use to pay his or her increased insurance premium does not address the root cause of the alleged *bad driving*. Additionally, since the issue isn't really resolved, poor driving may recur, leading to both financial difficulties and, worse yet, endangering health and safety.

As a result, when people rush to have trachea tissue-cutting surgery to treat their snoring, they may be ignoring the true root cause, which could be related to diet, sleep position, jaw or tongue dysfunction, lifestyle, genetics, or be an indication of a more serious health problem; an indication that could be dangerously suppressed (at least temporarily) following a seemingly successful surgery.

Surgery is like handing these bad drivers $500 in cash as an easy, on-the-spot cure for snoring. Although it may seem to be the answer to their problem, for many people, it will just be a short-term cure, hiding other underlying issues that might later result in serious repercussions, such as sleep apnea.

Reasons to refuse surgery for snoring surgery is often recommended as the first and only treatment for snoring. Many times, surgery is the first and only option available for treating a variety of illnesses. Snoring is an exception to this. Even while surgery has the potential to save lives and reduce suffering, there are additional expenses to consider. There is a plethora of reasons why surgery should not be considered due to the hazards connected with surgery, which include the following:

- Cosmetic effects after surgery
- An infection
- Inflammation and scar tissue

- Expensive postoperative treatments

- A lengthy recovery processes

- Expensive medications to treat swelling and relieve discomfort

- Potential for harm to speech and voice tone

- Swallowing difficulties

- Potential bleeding and seepage from the wound

- possibility of discomfortingly dry mouth

- The potential for excruciating earache

Overview of Surgical Procedures for Snoring

While surgery is a life-saving technique that has saved many lives, there is now a surgical treatment available for almost anything. Some of these processes may be unneeded and pointless. Surgery is not always a certain fix for issues with snoring in particular. Anyone who deals with snoring, whether directly or indirectly, must be aware of this when trying to find a solution.

The typical surgical solutions for snoring are discussed in the examples below, along with how they might let the patient down. The surgical operation's name, intended use, and—most importantly—the many negative consequences that have been attributed to each particular surgery are all stated in these cases.
The issues listed as a result of the various surgical techniques are grave.

The patient may have to deal with these issues after having snoring surgery, and they range from financial difficulties to long-term or permanent issues.

When you contemplate the issues that each of these procedures is truly intended to solve, it might be a complete turnoff. When there are so many additional possibilities accessible and linked to them, the cumulative impacts are something to be taken seriously. Once more, this is the reason why, if at all, surgery should typically only be considered as a last option.

There are additional hazards that are a part of any surgical treatment, but these other sorts of difficulties cannot be compared to the distinct collection of concerns that snoring generates and the various surgeries intended to address snoring. These risks are particular to surgical procedures for snoring. For instance, cost is always a concern, but it should be considered for a problem like snoring, while a problem like cancer or a failing organ requires spending money to prolong and enhance life. Anaesthesia carries another danger.

Being placed under anaesthesia during surgery is not always the case, but it is for any kind of serious operation. This would be necessary if you wanted to have surgery for your snoring, and anaesthetic has been known to cause difficulties, if not death, in certain cases.

Treatment Procedure

Tracheostomy

Make a hole in the trachea (sometimes this is called a tracheotomy). Nasal secretions may obstruct airways and cause breathing problems. UPPP (Uvulopalatopharyngoplasty) expands the airway and stops snoring. It is irritating to tissues and may cause scarring;

- o Cost-prohibitive, would necessitate another surgery if the blockage recurred, infection after surgery, and potential speech problems
- o increased chance of bleeding or swallowing issues
- o ineffective for treating sleep apnea

LAUP (Laser Assisted Uvuloplasty):

without removing the tonsils or lateral tissues, uses lasers to remove the uvula and obstructing tissues.

Dry mouth, changes in voice (to be avoided by those who depend on their voice for a living!), ear pain, an unpredictable success rate, and dry mouth can conceal deeper issues and/or cause new complications.

CAPSO (Cautery-Assisted Palatal Stiffening Operation)

Removes the mucosa along the uvula and burns the palate to stiffen it against vibration. Pain and discomfort following surgery Currently, we are in the testing phase (unproven).

price it is impossible to anticipate whether surgery will be successful.

In addition to these instances, novel snore-specific surgical procedures including somnoplasty and snoreplasty have been created. These treatments are brand-new and have not yet been shown to have any sort of consistent success rate. In addition, it is unknown if these types of snoring surgeries will have any long-term side effects.

Surgery is generally a very beneficial thing, but this does not indicate that it is the best course of action for treating snoring problems. To be clear, there are situations in which surgery is the best option for a person who snores, and the beneficial impacts are just as noticeable as the bad ones were when snoring was causing sleep deprivation and all the associated poor health conditions and mental states.

Fortunately, there are alternative choices. There are several non-surgical solutions for snoring; some of these solutions have been used for a while, while others are more recent. The bulk of relief from snoring comes from these less drastic measures to stop it. We will now look at some of the alternative techniques that many individuals use successfully to help themselves and others around them fall asleep and feel wonderful.

This page was left blank intentionally

CHAPTER THREE

Alternatives to Surgery for Snoring

We have already discussed the surgical aspects of snoring, the risks, and the procedures; now, let's focus on the more popular methods for treating snoring. The non-surgical treatments for treating snoring may be divided into many categories, including medications, equipment and gadgets, dietary and activity modifications, sleeping patterns, and alternative snoring therapy methods.

Depending on the underlying cause of the snoring and knowing what that underlying cause is, any of these methods can be successfully applied.

This may require a combination of approaches, and it will undoubtedly require observation of the effects of these measures on the snoring issue itself in order to estimate how much relief results.

Medicines: Prescribed medications may often provide relief from the snoring nightmare. Drugs are given to stop snoring by carrying out the following actions:

- o Spread the nasal airway out.
- o Boost your breathing energy.
- o Preventing deep R.E.M.
- o Sleep (rapid eye movement)

Sleep is essential for R.E.M. The body regains energy while the mind is able to remain alert and healthy throughout a deep sleep. In order to prevent the throat from relaxing too much and to maintain the airway clear and free of blockage, the function of these snore-related medicines is to restrict the depths to which the body may relax while in this condition, which results in relief from snoring. These drugs essentially have the opposite impact from what occurs when someone consumes too much alcohol or takes a sedative. These activities can cause an individual to become more relaxed than usual and exacerbate an existing snoring issue or cause someone who does not typically snore to start doing so.

Pharmacies provide over-the-counter medications designed particularly to cleanse nasal sinuses and airways. These medications are used to treat cold and flu symptoms, but since they also include decongestive and antihistamine qualities, they are also helpful for snorers. Saline sprays are included in the same category because they are offered in pharmacies as well.

These sprays are just salt water used to keep sinuses and other tissues around the air passages wet in an attempt to lessen or stop vibration and, in turn, snoring.

They are not restricted drugs.

Devices for Snoring People may deal with their snoring by using a variety of devices that are available. These items progress from the most basic to the most complex. The majority of these are available at your neighbourhood pharmacy, online, and through catalogues.

The following are the top-selling and most potent snore remedies;

The Pillow of Sandler

This device, which bears the name of the pillow's creator, forces the user to sleep on their side, which stops snoring. This often encourages closing your mouth as you sleep, which lessens vibration and eliminates any snoring.

A snooze balls

Numerous people have used this efficient device since it was created in the early 1900s to stop snoring by sleeping on their side. On the back of a pair of pyjamas, there is a pouch where the Snore Ball is placed. The gadget makes rolling onto one's back from sleeping on one's side very unpleasant, causing the user to return to sleeping on one's side instead of on one's back, which is the position in which most individuals snore.

Any ball that makes lying on one's back uncomfortable enough to prevent snoring may be used as a Snore Ball. As a habit develops over time, the ball becomes unneeded.

Monitor for Sleep Position

This technological innovation essentially achieves the same result in a different way. The sleep position monitor starts to beep when a person lies on their back, which is when snoring occurs, as opposed to causing physical discomfort. Others may find the beeping annoying, but the objective is that this gadget encourages the development of new sleeping habits.

Anyone who has experienced someone snoring can put up with a little beeping while the issue is being fixed. The individual will cease snoring if they discover a more comfortable sleeping position, and eventually the beeping won't be a problem. In time, it's possible that the sleep position monitor won't be required either.

Narcotic strips

This is a simple yet very powerful gadget that has gained popularity among many individuals. The idea is straightforward: Widen the nostrils to facilitate breathing. The tool is made up of an adhesive substance and a springy plastic strip. At night, the strip is worn, and in the morning, it is removed.

Numerous athletes from various sports use the strips because they maximize breathing through the nose.

Since there is no medicine involved, anyone can use this over-the-counter treatment. By breathing more easily and recharging their bodies with more oxygen, even those who don't snore are utilizing these strategies to obtain better, more peaceful sleep.

Narcotic Dilators

Nasal dilators, which differ slightly from nasal strips in how they work, provide the same relief as nasal strips by widening the nostrils to make breathing easier. This type of device is actually a steel or plastic coil inserted into the nostrils before bed. The effect is easier breathing and less snoring.

Mouth sprays

This is yet another approach to stopping snoring. To lessen or completely eliminate vibration, a simple spray at the back of the throat keeps the tissues well-lubricated. This is comparable to a saline spray, but unlike a saline spray, it contains specialized oils rather than just salt water. When used properly, throat sprays are another easy, affordable, and effective way to stop snoring. Overuse of throat sprays can irritate the throat and then actually cause snoring. If an over-the-counter spray is not good enough, a doctor can prescribe a more effective version of the same implement.

Stops Snoring

The purpose of the snore stopper is to halt snoring by creating a negative connection with it while the user is sleeping. When snoring is detected, the device, which can be worn on the wrist or arm, sends the snorer a brief electric shock to get them to stop. Another version really causes the tongue muscles to tighten, which opens the airway, making it easier to breathe, and consequently stops snoring.

Snoring Appliances: Snoring appliances are put within the mouth to directly impact or alter the components of the mouth to eliminate snoring. These work to adjust the tongue, jaw, and palate in some combination to reduce snoring and offer better slumber.

Oral Appliances: These kits of equipment are often created by medical and dentistry experts to address the snoring issue. They go by a variety of names, like The Equalizer and The Silencer. These devices work to stop snoring by influencing three fundamental aspects of the mouth, these are:

- o Closing the mouth to prevent snoring by stopping the trachea from vibrating.
- o Maintaining a forward-facing jaw position helps prevent the tongue from slipping back and obstructing the airway.
- o Increasing airway opening to improve breathing and stop snoring.

Devices for Retaining the Tongue

This sort of equipment primarily targets the tongue. The impact of this device maintains the tongue forward by employing suction to instruct the tongue not to lie back across the airway. This improves airflow, making breathing simpler and reducing the vibration that contributes to snoring.

Although a tongue retainer may not be the most comfortable alternative, it is a very successful one for those who cannot or will not sleep on their side.

Appliances for Mandibular Advancement

The acronym MAA refers to a splint-style appliance that functions somewhat similarly to a mouth guard worn by athletes. This prevents the jaw from sliding back and causing an obstruction that causes snoring. It also keeps the jaw frozen in place. These must be individually moulded by a dentist and may be pricey, but they are an excellent way to stop snoring.

Dr. Thronton developed the Silencer, a well-known example of this kind of tool, in the 1990s. This option is pricey, but for good reason—it is adjustable and occasionally made of titanium. These are frequently referred to as TAPs, and they function similarly to MAAs in that they advance the jaw to keep the airway open and stop snoring.

The Palate-Lifters

This device, sometimes known as lip shields or lip lifters, strengthens the palate to prevent vibrations that may otherwise cause snoring. Although there isn't yet a certain consensus on the effectiveness of this kind of equipment, this is a possibility to take into account.

Positive airway pressure that is constant

This device is particularly designed to address sleep apnea. It functions similarly to an oxygen mask. The mask is worn on the face or over the nose and maintains what is termed "positive pressure" in the airway, which prevents the collapse of tissue and eases breathing to the point of managing one's blood pressure while sleeping.

Lifestyles and Snoring—Diet Allergies

Allergies have been related to snoring, but since there are so many allergens, and each person is different, it is up to the individual to watch when they are snoring and what they are allergic to. Any allergic response, whether it be to food or a pet, may cause snoring, so if you have allergies, you should be aware of them and take the necessary precautions to manage them.

Weight If you snore and are overweight, you can guarantee that your obesity is at least partially to blame for your snoring. Better health outcomes from weight loss include less snoring and better sleep. This has to do with your food and eating routine, so if you get in shape, you could completely stop snoring.

Eating Patterns Some foods, such as dairy, fried meals, junk food, and sweets, promote congestion. If you snore, your food undoubtedly has something to do with it. Eating a healthy diet may enhance your health as well as lessen, if not completely relieve, any snoring. There are meals that are considered healthy for people who snore and are mostly made up of leafy greens.

Clean Living Your behaviours may impact whether or not you snore. Healthy habits actually prevent snoring. Drinking and taking sleeping aids are known to make people snore; use these things sparingly. If you smoke and snore, it's likely that quitting will improve your sleep quality because you won't snore. Caffeine has been linked to respiratory difficulties, so limit your consumption to a minimum.

Lifestyles and Snoring: Exercise

Exercise in general is healthy for the body and helps to obtain more peaceful sleep. Healthy behaviours can be avoided to lessen snoring, but there are snoring-specific exercises one may undertake.

Throat Workout Toning the muscles of the throat may substantially enhance the respiratory process while sleeping, thereby aiding with snoring if not removing it all together. There are a few ways to work the snoring-related muscles. For up to five minutes, you can firmly hold a pencil between your teeth. Building jaw strength involves applying moderate pressure to the chin for a short period of time.

The tongue is strengthened by pressing the tip firmly against the lower front teeth. You may do these exercises anywhere, at any time. These shouldn't hurt, and the more often you do them, the better the results you'll get.

Sleep Factors One needs to consider the way in which one sleeps and how that affects the way one breathes at night. Sleeping on your back promotes snoring, but having a good pillow or sleeping with something under your chin can help to stop snoring. Anything to keep the mouth shut during sleep is a tremendous benefit. Your sleep environment also plays a role in snoring.

A humidifier will assist in keeping the throat and sinuses moist, and having the room as dark and quiet as possible helps to minimize tension and relax the person sleeping to the point where breathing becomes easier. Alternatives to snoring therapy Here are some alternative ways one may attempt when dealing with snoring; some have been around for some time because of how beneficial they have been in controlling snoring. a warm drink before bed; herbal tea may actually help decrease snoring. Numerous snorers have found great relief using breathing exercises and relaxation techniques like Tai Chi and Yoga.

Other methods of unwinding include massages, meditation, and even just listening to relaxing music. Snoring can be treated in a variety of ways with homeopathic remedies as well. These include items like Y-Snore and Snore Stop. Homeopathic options aim to accomplish the same goal in several methods, such as by clearing nasal and throat obstructions or lubricating the joints using natural ingredients.

Popular in China, magnetic therapy can reduce snoring by influencing the nerves in the nose. Magnets can be applied all over the body to get results that reduce snoring problems. This applies even to weight reduction, which might in turn impact snoring. Even hypnosis has been used to help reduce snoring by some; however, many are wary of this method since it is not recognized as a viable treatment for snoring. Other, more unconventional treatments rely on the healing properties of light, colour, or, in some cases, gems and crystals.

The effectiveness of these latter examples has not yet been proven by science or medicine, but the placebo effect may still occur. So long as the goal is to stop snoring, any method can

be tried and tested to see if it works for a
particular person.